Sex–Let's Talk About Sex in a Christian Bed:

Experiencing a Taste of Heaven Together

Dr. Nadine Wong

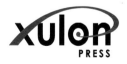

xulon
PRESS

Sex - Let's Talk About Sex in a Christian Bed: Experiencing a Taste of Heaven Together
by Dr. Nadine Wong

Printed in the United States of America.

ISBN 9781498498913

www.xulonpress.com

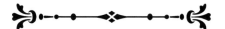

This book is dedicated to my Lord and Savior, Jesus Christ, who has renewed my mind spiritual and physically, and in science.

Table of Contents

Introduction

There are many misconceptions in some Christian circles about sex. As a therapist who, for over 10 years, specializes in Single, Family, Marriage, Nutrition and Sex Therapy, I have heard everything from the notion that sex is ONLY for procreation, to perceptions that Christians do not or should not have sexual desires or that Christians do not desire to have great sex. Nothing could be further from the truth.

Sex for the Christian actually should be a glorious interaction, because sex in a covenant relationship, or marriage between a man and a woman, is really an act of worship. It is the epitome of the fulfillment of

God's intent that 'two become one' (Matthew 19:5). That's why both sex and intimacy are essential pillars in a covenant relationship. And to experience strong sex, in which both partners 'enjoy a taste of heaven', requires strong communication between the man and the woman.

Everyone has a personal viewpoint regarding sex and having great sex, even from a Christian perspective. *Let's Talk Sex in a Christian Bed* is an educational handbook for single people in-waiting and married couples who wish to ignite the fire of experiencing strong sex in their union. With permission, I've shared a few of my client's stories who have a strong Christian faith but struggled with various sexual issues to help provide clarity on some of the topics shared.

This book lays a solid foundation to understand and prepare well for this act of worship in marriage and provides rarely discussed insights and keys to a healthy, vibrant and fulfilling union.

Dr. Nadine Wong

CEO, Alabaster Wellness Clinic

Chapter One

What is Sex?

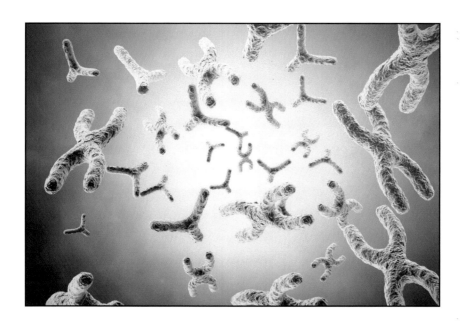

In preaching the gospel, there are very few sermons that openly speak of the scientific demonstration of the power of God as it pertains to sex in the Christian bed. Many lay church leaders shy away from talking about this topic publicly and, in extreme cases, privately causing many marriages within the church to quietly flounder from sexual dysfunction, and too many Christian singles are left without proper guidance to navigate their emotions and sexual urges in a wholesome manner.

Let's look at the science behind sex as our starting point to help us better understand what it is and debunk some of the mysteries and misconceptions about the normalcy of sex that trip some Christian singles and married couples.

What is sex?

Sex is both an internal and external process. It is more mental than physical. Someone for example, who is distracted with thoughts of work, children or some other responsibility will find it difficult to fully engage and enjoy oneness with their spouse during sex. Because sex requires both mental and physical participation, a genuine syncopated taste of heaven–strong sex–is more difficult to achieve when one or both partners have mentally checked out!

At the scientific level, sex is a metabolism of an involuntary reaction of chemicals in maintaining the living state of cells and their organisms. The origin of sex begins from within a cell unit. This means that sex is the anatomy and physiology of structures and their forms, and the function of their parts. Allow me to walk you through this amazing tripartite ecology.

The levels of organization within the human body are composed of chemical substances. These substances are composed of tiny invisible particles called atoms. Atoms commonly bind together to form larger particles called molecules. Molecules combined together to form larger molecule organelles that carry on specific activities. Within the organelles are compositions of chemicals including proteins, carbohydrates, fats, and DNA information.

Organelles combine to form cells that contain DNA information. Cells are structured layers with common functions. A group of cells form a tissue. Groups of unlike tissues form organs with specialized functions that operate as an organ system. An organ system creates a complete organism, known as functioning human systems.

God so intricately and purposefully designed us and he is pleased with how he has created us (Genesis 1:27, 31). David recognized this when he declared, "I praise you because I am fearfully and wonderfully made..." (Ps 139:14). Laying the scientific foundation of sex gives light to the fact that sex is created by God; therefore, the desire for sex is a normal chemical reaction within the human body; and mankind needs sex.

Just as money is not the root of all evil, sex in and of itself is not a sin. Sex is a scientific cycle from which we each originate. Whether we are conceived by natural or artificial insemination, human development begins with production from the sex organs.

Sex is a natural biological function created in every human being by God. This biological function does not cease to exist when you make a vow to follow God. The desire for sex is also not an unnatural inclination or an evil to be rebuked or a feeling to be ashamed. Rather it is a metabolic interaction that, like any other desire, is mediated by our exercise of mental control. That's why when the Bible teaches that a Christian should renew their mind (Romans 12:2, Ephesians 4:23) about sex and other behaviors, it is this process that separates them from the unbeliever. As we learn, understand and align with and apply God's principles we are empowered to honor his will for us even as it pertains to sex.

Chapter 2

Natural Desire of Sex

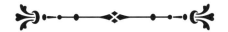

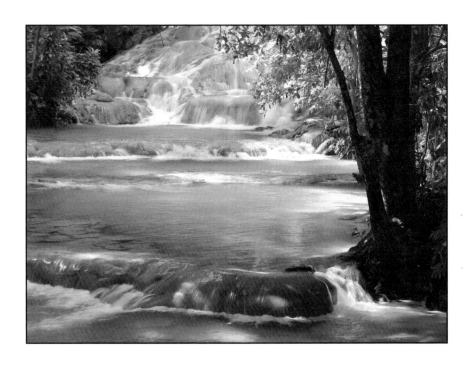

A *35-year old Christian female was trying to live a godly life and chose to abstained from sex when she met and fell in love with a Christian man. They soon became inseparable. She said that whenever they held hands it was as if her blood 'literally' boiled. "One day I smelled his cologne and before we knew it, we were engrossed in passionate love making," she lamented. Ashamed that she gave into this desire, she turned in confidence to a female church leader who without hesitation chastised her and disassociated from her. Confused by her desires and the quandary of emotions that tormented her, she became angry with the spiritual leader, inadvertently with God, and left the church.*

In and outside my practice, I have heard of many similar instances in which individuals have left their church because they struggled with their sexual desires and believed there was no genuine or empathic help.

In another instance a young man told of being sexually aroused in church during service. He admitted that every time he sat behind certain sisters he could not help himself. "Their clothes hugged their fearfully and wonderfully made curves, hints of their delicate lacy under garments often peek over their gluteal maximus or butts crack. Sometimes seeing all that," he explained "was inadvertently stimulating." So, for his own salvation, he promoted himself to sit in the front row to avoid any unnecessary distraction.

What drives the desire for sex?

The struggle with sexual desire for both females and males, as illustrated in the story above, is common within Christian communities. What they each experience in arousal and desire is a natural chemical process within the human body. Allow me to explain.

The desire of sex is regulated through the metabolism of two glands: the endocrine gland and the exocrine gland.

The endocrine gland transports substances, regulates water, electrolyte balance, and blood pressure by controlling the chemical reactions and also contributes to growth, reproduction, and development.

The exocrine gland has duct-like structures that transports substances in the skin, for example sweat and sebaceous oils.

Sex is a hormonal biochemical secretion, which stimulates changes by targeting cells that affect the function of other cells. Other cells are affected by altering the metabolic processes of an enzyme necessary for the synthesizing of substances, or are chemically altered when being transported through the cell membranes. In order for this transportation to take place the hormones bind to specific receptors that affect other cells.

Consequently, the desire to have sex is the effects of the metabolism of the cell communicating with specific receptors that receive messages. The messages are intercepted by the gland in the brain, called the hypothalamus, which interprets sight, sound, smell, taste, or touch. These cellular interactions result in causing a reaction to carry out the metabolic process of the physical interaction of sex and hence activates the desire for sex, as the woman and man at the beginning of this chapter experienced. Regulating this chemical reaction is a fortitude of mental control that strengthens with the renewing of the mind through God's word.

Chapter 3

Preparation for Sex

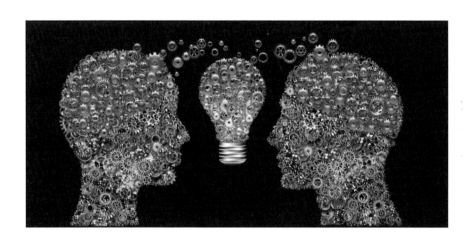

A woman I know had been preparing herself for marriage for many years. She struggled with her weight and eventually had weight loss surgery. She finally met and married a wonderful man; however, despite her remodeled body she struggled in her marriage with intimacy. She could not receive or accept her husband's compliments. She just could not see herself as the 'Queen' he adored, loved and desired; because in her mind she still perceived herself as unattractive.

I share her story because the preparation for sex is more mental than physical. It is vitally important for one to be confident as described by God, whose Word validates your body aesthetic. When you see yourself as God sees you, you can rejoice, like David, in knowing that you are fearfully and wonderfully made (Psalm 139:14). You can foster a healthy body image by letting the Word of God transform your mind. The irritation of any physical imperfections will pale as you gain wisdom, knowledge and understanding (Daniel 1:4).

In this we can appreciate the Bible verse, "… perfect love casts out all fears…" (1 John 4:18) and "Love covers the multitude of all sin *[imperfection]*" (1 Peter 4:8). Note in this context, sin is used as imperfection. Once you accept you and your spouse's imperfections, you can both be free to be naked and unashamed (Genesis 2:25). Such confidence will remove the hindrance of insecurity from the altar of worship to God and to the perfect unity in husband and wife knowing each other and becoming one.

Preparing for sex also requires physical skills in both men and women. Ladies, this is especially true to strengthen devoid muscles that can easily become bruised through penetration, or as it is biblically termed when "knowing" your husband. Men, it is not uncommon to experience pre-ejaculation until your mental stamina builds.

The physical preparation for sex, therefore, has to be kinetic. You must physically exercise to build stamina. Let me caution and stress that building up your large muscles, by working out in the gym, is not an indication of strong endurance when it comes to performing sex. Although engaging only in weight training results in big, tight muscles, yet you may not have the mental stamina to endure sexual kinetic. Therefore, do not be concerned solely with size.

I recommend taking a simple physical test as a guide of each other's sexual endurance. Walk up ten flights of stairs together. Two things will happen; you will arrive at the top together or one person will arrive before the other. If you arrive three or more steps ahead of your spouse, then your stamina is greater. You then need to be patient with the other person to get to your level. The same principle can be applied to sexual stamina and reaching an orgasm. If there is any disparity between the sexual dexterity of husband and wife, apply patience until your stamina level is the same and to taste heaven together.

Woman: if you are a virgin, which by definition is a person who has never had sexual intercourse or known a man, or if you have abstained from all forms of sexual self-gratification, it is likely that on your wedding night you may experience a level of discomfort or light bleeding.

Man: if you are a virgin, which by definition is a person who has never had penetrative sexual intercourse with or known a woman or if you have abstained from all forms of sexual self-gratification, don't be embarrassed if your endurance lasts only uncontrolled seconds, at least at the first attempt. That's normal! These experiences are attributed to unused kinetic mental muscles. As illustrated in the example of the stairs test, this is where you must exercise patience with each other and build your stamina together so that you can be in unity and taste heaven together!

Now let's get back to the science of sex to understand what occurs within the body in preparation for sex. A woman's vaginal walls are layers of various types of elastic tissue and soft muscles. Upon arousal, the linings will secrete lubricants as the hypothalamus is activated and sends out messages to the sexual glands that prepare the body for sex. Hence, intensify the sensation you feel during sex. During sexual penetration, vaginal secretion will reduce most discomfort. Secreted lubrication will brace the thrust of a man's penis, even though initially there will be some level of discomfort from the unused muscles.

Wives, sex is a need your husband MUST have fulfilled. A woman's curvy vagina is naturally molded to contour the beam of a penis. The essential beam, his penis, is a symbol of dominance more than any other human organ. When a man is stimulated, his penis will become erected and, in some cases, sometimes tripled in size; an average of nine inches in length and five inches in width.

Having sex and breathing is synergetic. Breathing will appease and relax the mind. It will enhance stamina, and minimize any need to over exert with physical kinetic that causes lengthen to short stop. "Breathe to prolong life." (Genesis 2:7). So, let your breathing pattern be your guide. The more you control your breathing, the more it will systemically prolong endurance. Don't hyperventilate! Timing the thrust in penetration can both reduce pain for a woman and pre-ejaculation in a man, and result in husband and wife having an organism or tasting heaven together.

As mentioned previously, be fully present when you are engaging in intercourse with your spouse. Remember that sex is more mental than physical. Allow your senses to be your guide to access your mental stamina. Otherwise, the mind can easily stray into the subconscious to access thoughts or wonder to last week's presentation, or finances, or past failures or futurist life goals. Guard your mind. Be present and enjoy the experience. When you do, the flood gates of sexual hormones are released. As the arousal signals transmit to the physical body, if you are not mentally present, it will gallop in a non-rhythmic manner. This will delay tasting heaven together.

Chapter 4

Wife Preparing for Sex with Her Husband: The Top Three Stimuli for Men

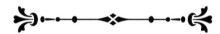

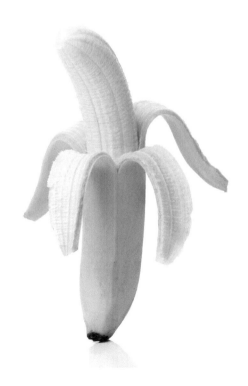

We conducted an informal study to identify the most important stimuli for men and women. In separate random surveys, we asked both men and women to provide the characteristics in their spouse that made having sex more desirous and enjoyable. The top three responses may surprise you. Men prize hygiene; confidence–body imagine; and the tie-breaker, submission or communication. To this same question, women said what they valued most from men were: tenderness, patience and communication.

Hygiene–Men will NOT compromise on hygiene! The French coins the vaginal fragrance as 'cassolette'. The cassolette is the natural odor or perfume of a carefully clean woman. A woman's natural fragrance or her pheromone, to some men can be her greatest sexual asset. Men will use hygiene fragrance, like that of a hunter who zooms in on his next delightful meal, or his wife floral.

Other popular hygiene preferences for men are: groomed to zero pubic hair, notification on menstrual cycle, and in some cases, meticulous shower and toilet habits. These preferences intensify a man's hunting skills. Even in the wild, animals use this technique to ignore sick or wounded prey animals.

Confidence–Men typically use their senses to detect how confident you are. They say the more confident you are with self-imagine, the more enjoyable sex is for them. Ladies, to ensure an enjoyable experience, relax as he leads. Flow with him. Give and receive each other as a gift. This harmony of the two becoming one is very endearing. It channels a sense of controlled sexual submission through the body once it is processed as sexual confidence and not as arrogance. You are a gift to your husband! And your confidence in engaging with him is a fruit of that gift.

You are good gift to him from God, do not become like the fig tree that was cursed to die, simply because it did not bear any fruit or gifts of fruits (Mark 11:12-14).

Communication–Outside of sex, men are not credited to be great communicators. To locate keys to unlock his heaven, be sensitive to his non-verbal cues. Chose the appropriate time, preferable not during sex (least he interprets it as emasculation), to share your likes and dislikes of his sexual performances. Remember, strong communication facilitates strong sex. Be mindful also that your husband wants to know how he can please you, as doing so pleases him. So, listen and you may accomplish harmonious flow where you are ready to receive him under the average 15 minutes!! When you know what each other equates as strong sex and make that a priority, sex becomes a most powerful experience.

Chapter 5

Husband Preparing for Sex with His Wife: The Top Three Stimuli for Women

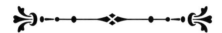

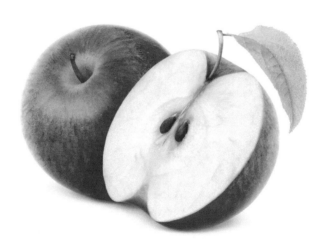

Naturally, men are hunters. Hunters use the left side of their brain to make practical and precise decisions. Therefore, it is quite natural for a man to take the lead in everything including initiating sex. This has it strengths, but men keep in mind that without including communication, patience, and tenderness, your wife may have a challenging time harmonizing with you during sex. Become a master in these three stimuli that women prize, above all else, for experiencing strong sex.

Tenderness–Like a man's body there are obvious signs that confirm your wife's readiness for penetration. Her pupils will dilate, breast and nipples become firm, clitoris becomes erected and warm vaginal lubrication will involuntarily discharge with her distinct pheromone. To help her experience strong sex, demonstrate tenderness not excitement. Approach her with gentle, yet firm touches slowly to avoid bruising or laceration to her sex organs. Be mindful that seconds after a woman climaxes, her sexual organs are most sensitive. That's the time to be most tender, if she can still receive your touch.

Patience–Always demonstrate patience! Only if a woman lets you in can there be harmony between you. Patience takes experience. It requires a commitment of time and work. But the reward is priceless. To be harmonious with your wife becomes your second skin over time. To reduce frustration in this endeavor, make this note to self; on an average a woman takes 15 minutes to completely become harmonious to receive all of your manhood. Therefore, find one hundred ways to orchestrate her syncopation that will reduce the preparation time from 15 minutes to 15 seconds!

Communication–Women almost certainly use their sense of hearing more than other senses to get into a sexual mood. Therefore, men be ready to express yourself! But first prepare. Ask her questions. Do not assume anything. The importance of communication before sex is to gather information to prolong your 'happily ever after'.

Be honest with your wife about any previous sexual experiences, and openly discuss together both your sexual likes and dislikes. Ask follow-up questions, such as menstrual cycle, for you do not want an unscheduled guest, especially on your honeymoon. Share realistic fantasies, perhaps how to become one such as in the shower, or anoint bodies with olive oil, or adorn the bed with fresh rose petals, or set the mood with ambient lights or mirrors on the ceiling. Create an atmosphere to arouse a sexual encounter with stimulants you both will enjoy. Speak each other's language, play syncopating music as you set the mood and tone to taste heaven together. Note: Amazing Grace, on record has never influenced anyone to have sex!

Chapter 6

Playful Continuous Sex

❧⟩•⸱•⸱•❖•⸱•⟨❧

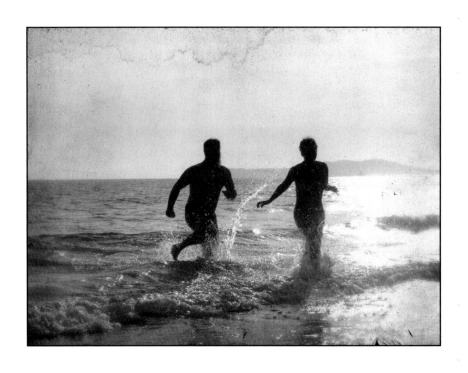

During playtime, the body naturally replenishes, repairs, and releases endorphins, or happy chemical hormones to balance the biological immune system. This is the perfect opportunity for partners to collect sexual data for the next sexual experience. It is also the perfect time to relax, breathe, laugh out loud, and become as curious with playfulness, as a child, to each other.

Playtime can be created from anything. Take items from the scriptures in the Book of Song of Solomon for example, to create a platter: nectar, honey, apple, rose, savory textures, grapes, lily of the valley, aloes, various flowers, or spices of saffron, cinnamon, frankincense, and chief spices. Challenge each other in a simple task such as a game of cards or a board game. At the end of the game, let the winner request of their partner anything from the platter. Be creative. Let your request be made known to your partner on "How" you desire to be served.

Playtime can be accomplished with simple notes or surprises. I once heard of a couple who collected cultural items and stored them in small gift boxes. Their objective was to incorporate diversity and fantasy. They included various cultural spices that non-verbally indicated the choice of meal for date night. Other items you could include in the boxes include: lingerie with a card or notes of adoring yet stimulating words, your partner's favorite dessert, ticket to their favorite game or show, or just simple treasure hunt steps with stimulating results that complete covenant trust and strength in the relationship.

The playground can be your oyster! Be creative in the shower, kitchen, car, or park, if you're both adventurous. Schedule time to send suggestive notes or video messages to each other on the job. Once again, playtime is among partners only, not children or with any outside distractions.

Chapter 7

Nutrition and Sex

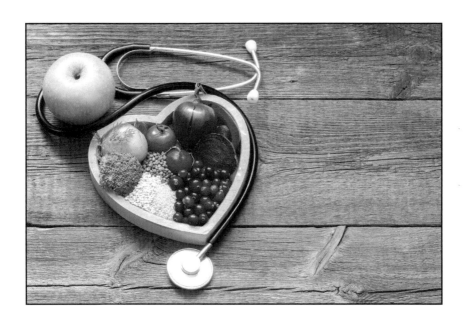

A wife refused to have sex with her husband for months. Her excuse was that her menstrual cycle never stopped. To avoid hurting her husband's feelings she refrained from communicating to him the real issue which was that, "His semen smelt like raw sewage". Now, raw sewage has it prefect place in a bio-ecology environment, but not during sex.*

You may have heard it said that you are what you eat! Everything sweet, savory, starchy, or spicy, or even medication, will convert itself and have an adverse effect on your stamina or produce a questionable taste or unpleasant body odor. The lack of exercise can also result in a strong and pungent pheromone that discourages an alluring partner. Many a partner can relate to being turned off by unpleasant body odors. This can be quite off-putting and negatively impact intimacy with your spouse, as illustrated in the encounter of the wife at the beginning of this chapter.

Food is as important to the body as oil is to the efficient running of an engine. The body needs to be maintained after a few 'thousand miles' to sustain your heart, mind, balance body odor and your physical wellbeing.

Foods that are most beneficial to your health are fresh pulps protein, dark greens, vibrant fruits, grains of starch with fresh herbs, and salt for flavor. An overly salty or sugary diet has the ability to dehydrate the body's cells that cause an abnormal blood pressure that result in poor stamina.

Reduce consistent consumption of spicy meals such as tomatoes, hot peppers, or garlic, as these herbs will transport within the cellular fluid lysosome and generate unpleasant body odors. The lysosome is a decomposing enzyme that breaks down protein, fats and starches that secrete into the lymphatic system. The lymphatic system or the drainage system in males drains through semen, and in women it drains through the vaginal secretion and releases an unattractive odor.

Simple foods that are high in antioxidants maintain and increase pheromone. Antioxidants are enzymes that have the ability to help the body's immune system fight free radicals or aliments that can result in sluggish or unbalanced hormones and consequently, affect sexual appetite. Dark greens such as kale, spinach, spirulina, or flavonoid rich fruits such as berries, pineapple, cranberry and citrus naturally detoxify the lymphatic system and body secretion. Through perspiration, a process of sweating, pores of the skin cells excrete oils. The oils attract itself to either unsaturated oils with an alluring fragrance, or to saturated oils that result in a rancid deficient scent.

Conclusion

Sex is Life

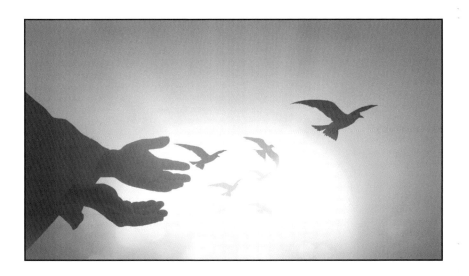

S ex is a need. The art of sex is a natural biological function that can be described as the gateway to heaven. And to experience an orgasm is to taste a piece of heaven. Sometimes the journey will have its obstacles and can lead to an unpleasant outcome. However, to marry which is a mature decision, demands work.

As you become one, that is knowing your partner through sexual intercourse, it is the first marriage covenant of worship unto God (Mark 10:8). Sex is a transfer of honor through worship to God, the author of science and the One who created the human anatomy and physiology, and who through his spirit gave us his breathe of life (Genesis 2:7).

Once there is an agreement between partners, be creative in how you honor and please each other. Be purposeful to communicate with each other, be playful and open to explore different sexual positions and to

create new levels of pleasure that will produce unified orgasm.

As openly as sin is ministered from the
pulpit, sex should be ministered with the
same thrust of skills in wisdom, cunning in
knowledge, and an understanding of God's
scientific skills to edify, instruct and guide
the believer's life. The messages from the
pulpit must be balanced to demonstrate
that sex has its purpose in life and is not
just to procreate a life.

The church should be of the same con-
viction, that sex outside of marriage is the
same sin as not having sex or not being
satisfied sexually in marriage. The reality
is there are more Christian couples who
have succumbed to public marriage, yet
sibling relationship in their bedroom. This
could result from a lack of anatomy and
physiology communication in pre-marital
counselling to decode sex as healthy and
not dirty.

It is my hope that *Let's Talk Sex in a Christian Bed* inspires healthy and informed conversations about sex. May Christian singles in waiting find relief from understanding the science behind sex and embrace the normalcy of what they experience in their bodies. And may more Christian couples be refreshed through the guidelines provided to have strong conversations which is vital to have strong sex and experience a taste of heaven together.

About the Author

Dr. Nadine Wong, PhD

Dr. Nadine Wong is a Clinical Psychotherapist, with a Doctorate in Integrative Medicine and Trichology (hair, scalp and their disorders). She is also the CEO for Alabaster Wellness Clinic, Developer of Alabaster Beauty Ointment, and founder of Alabaster Gates Children's Charity.

For more than 10 years, Dr. Wong has specialized in Single, Family, Marriage, Nutrition and Sex Therapy, Integrative Medicine, and developing and researching cosmetic beauty ointment products.

Dr. Wong's mandate is, through scientific research to validate health and for it to be viewed as one unit. The issues of mental health, application of cosmetics, and consumption of foods are a ramification as a result of exposure to products.

For more information visit www.alabasterwellness.com.